No Fads Just Facts

No Fads Just Facts

Never Give Up

Michael A. Bacigalupi

To order additional copies of this book, contact:
Xlibris Corporation
1-888-795-4274
www.Xlibris.com
Orders@Xlibris.com
52449

Contents

DEDICATION

I dedicate this book to my grandmother Julia (Mama Julia) Daniels. As a kid you never know what you learn until you grow up. Mama Julia did not care about what she would receive; she would just care what she could give. I have learned my compassion to everyone through her. She was so compassionate towards everyone. Grandma you are truly my Guardian Angel and I know God has you looking down on me and guiding me through life. Thank you so much for everything you did and continue to do for me. I will always love you and take your heart with me and instill them in my two kids.

For My Loving Family Debra, Caitlyn and Austin

Acknowledgements

I would like to thank God for the vision he has set for me and for opening my eyes when they were closed.

Thank you Debra for understanding that writing this book means so much to me and for all the sacrifices you made for me so I can achieve all my goals. I hope both of my kids, Caitlyn and Austin, will appreciate the hard work I went through to successfully accomplish what I set out to do.

To my parents Gary and Georgia Bacigalupi, you are the best . . . you continually help others before you help yourselves; you are both God's helpers. Both of you have touched my life and so many others you come in contact with. I love you both and thank you for all you have done for me and my family.

To my brother Tony Bacigalupi, I am so proud of you. You have overcome so much and seeing you pull out of it gives me strength; I wish you all the best. I love you bro.

No Fads, Just Facts

Sitting here reflecting on this journey takes me back to the beginning when I realized I didn't have the respect of my closest friends and co-workers. I saw a picture of myself at a company Christmas party in 2006. "Whoa"! I thought to myself, "that can't be me"! I then remember looking at myself in the mirror and asking "what have you done to yourself?" I didn't realize I had let myself go that bad. My weight was 236 lbs and at 5'6", that was considered extremely obese. It not only affected my personal life, but my professional life as well. I found it increasingly difficult to perform my everyday duties at work. That's not me; I am a very outgoing person with lots of energy but my body was telling me otherwise. One day I broke down after looking at that picture again; I was so angry, I called myself every name in the book. I knew I had to make a change; you know, find something that would motivate me to lose weight. Aside from the appearance, I knew I needed to get my blood pressure down to a healthy reading in order to live longer and see my kids grow up. I recall telling myself, "get your ass up and stop making excuses." And that's when I began . . . I started eating healthy and working out.

I played high school football and some college baseball so I knew my way around the gym. But when it came to a health program, I made many mistakes, including not giving any program I tried, long enough to work. I would try one program for about two or three weeks, get frustrated and move on to another program and do the very same thing over again.

Most sensible weight programs work, but you have to give it a reasonable amount of time. One mistake people (myself included) make is saying "there's not enough time". How often do we use that excuse? Quitting (or never beginning) is easy, and we use that phrase to justify quitting or to just not begin. If you don't overcome that excuse, you can't realize the gratification you feel when you begin and finish a program. When I finished my first program I felt I could accomplish anything.

I learned to set small attainable goals for myself so I can complete them and then move on to the next. In this book I will show you the program I used and then I will break it down for you into small goals.

Gaining the respect of my family and friends was motivation for me. When I started working out and getting stronger and leaner, my colleagues started joining me in the gym. That was the first time I remember inspiring someone, and let me tell you, that was a wonderful feeling. My decision to get in shape has sparked a trend in my workplace; I helped the company I work for implement a corporate wellness program. I can now honestly say I have gained the respect of my colleagues . . . they now come to me with their questions and asking for advice.

Another benefit of being fit is the positive affect it has in my professional world. I am now able to accomplish more physical work in a shorter period of time, providing more time to make more money for the company, which in turn, keeps the owners of the company I work for happy.

Here's a little information about what I do to put food on my family's table. I work for a chemical production company. This company manufactures chemicals for the water treatment industry. I won't bore you with specifics since this is a fitness book; in general, some of the blends we make require some heavy lifting in the process. There are times we need to put 1,200 or 2,200 lbs. (50 lbs. each bag) of a certain chemical. In the past, it would take me a long time to finish that certain blend. Today 2,200 lbs. of 50 lb. bags is nothing and I can finish in ten to fifteen minutes. That in turn helps the company because I can put more products out the door in a shorter amount of time.

So you can see staying fit helps you perform your daily tasks easier and with less stress. Working out and staying fit lowers stress during the day; that is a fact . . . so get out and burn some calories!

Chapter One

Why

How Long

Looking at my time frame, I would say my weight loss did not begin until after I committed to a program and stayed with it for around twelve weeks. There are many twelve-week programs out there but most of us look at that to be too long. I once had a client ask me, "What can I do to lose the most weight in the shortest amount of time?" I answered, "liposuction", that's the problem right there; we live in a fast food, fast-paced world. We expect instant results with no work involved. It took me about twelve weeks to lose 67 lbs but I didn't notice the weight dropping until around week six. That told me you need to give the program ample time to work. In the middle of week six I started studying to become a certified personal trainer. I wasn't going to rest until I started helping others. I was there before; walking the same path you are. Not someone who has never been fat before. You know the ones you see on TV infomercials promising you the world in as little as two weeks. Send me $49.95 and you could lose up to 10lbs a week. They know you feel miserable and they will take advantage of your low self esteem. Come on, you are smarter than that. Think about the satisfaction you will get when you lose weight that you work so hard to lose.

One thing you must realize, you have to commit to a life style change. I also said to myself, "okay, I am 35 years old. I have been putting junk in my body for over fifteen years, so now let's try to put only good food in from now on." It's not as hard as you think. I know will power is very hard to come by for some people; let's face it, if everyone had will power, we wouldn't have this type of problem. Will power was the hardest thing for me to attain, but I approached it like I approached my workout routine. So the "how long" question would be continuous . . . it's on-going.

After beginning, you should start to see some results after about four or five weeks. I always say, "If you can get past the first couple of weeks, then you should be on your way to a successful weight loss program." Like I said before, most people expect to see results after a couple of days. Just stay with it and soon enough, you will begin to see results. There are many challenges out on the market these days. I highly recommend you find one and start as soon as possible. As incentive, give yourself small rewards after you complete each week or segment. I will talk more about that when I talk about your program.

Research

Once I started working out and the gym became apart of my everyday routine, I researched weight loss and weight loss control because I wanted this to stay with me. I did not want to be one of those that lost 100 lbs just to gain 130 lbs after six months. I did not want to go back to where I came from. It doesn't mean anything if you gain it back. I see it as unfulfilled goals. So I started reading about weight loss and the proper gym techniques which inspired me to earn my Personal Trainer Certificate. The first thing I learned was any weight loss program is based on the principle that when the number of calories burned by a person in 24 hours is greater than the number of calories consumed, weight loss takes place in the individual. Wow! It can't be that easy. If it was that easy, then everyone should lose weight. Also, I did not know that 1 pound of fat is equal to 3500 calories. So for me to lose 1 lb, I would need to burn 3500 calories. Okay, now it's starting to get complicated. I can't burn 3500 calories, it would take too long. Yes, that is too long; weight loss takes too long, no wonder we all give up. I will get back to that later.

I learned the benefits of exercise and fitness. Correct and regular exercise result in a large number of benefits, not only to the body but also to the mind. It improves your mental outlook and your mood due to the release of chemicals called endorphins in the body . . . and let me tell you, it feels great. It improves general health, wards off diseases, and slows down the aging process. It helps you achieve a better body composition, lowers body fat and increases muscle. It improves the state of mind, promotes better mental health, and improves sleep. It also helps to avoid atrophy. Atrophy refers to the shrinkage of muscle as a result of little or no exercise. Extreme exercise leads to hypertrophy, which refers to the tissue and muscles gaining in strength due to over load. We will talk about those two terms later in the book. But research is very important when you begin a weight loss program. Anytime you begin something like this, you should research it first. Go to the library or go on-line. Learn about what you're doing and why you're doing it . . . you will be much more successful.

Setting Goals

When you begin your program, make sure you have set long-term and short-term goals. Short term goals will keep you on track to complete your long term goals. I also recommend creating small rewards for yourself after you complete each goal. Your weight loss goal should be no more than about two pounds per week. I suggest you reward yourself every two to three weeks; pick a gift you want and after you complete one goal get your gift. What I did was buy myself clothes that were too little . . . like pants. When I started my weight loss program I was in a size 38 pants. I bought a pair of 36 and 34 and now I wear a size 32. So my goal was to get into those jeans. Shirts also, I always wanted to wear fitted shirts from the Gap and I went from an extra large to a medium. And today I wear those shirts from the Gap. Clothing is only one example. I also gave my wife some incentive; I told her that if she loses a certain amount of weight, I will take her on a cruise. So you can see, as you reward yourself, you find the program not so hard to complete. I found that when I completed a certain part of the program that was incentive enough for me. But, I will tell you, it felt good to put those size 32 jeans on. Set realistic goals, goals you know you will be able to complete. Don't set unrealistic goals . . . you don't want to overwhelm yourself into discouragement. Unrealistic goals tend to make people give up too easy. The most popular goal is clothes. I think more people tend to want to get in that smaller size pants or shirts. So I recommend getting a smaller size pant and start losing. Good luck and remember it will start to come off if you stick to it. Make the life-long change, not the short term change.

I recall after about 10 weeks into my program, my energy level got so high that I started wanted to run long distances. I set more goals for myself. I did some research on local 5k events (3 miles . . . I can do that!). I had never run that far before. So I started running and a couple of months later, I entered and ran in my first 5k with a time of 33:40. This might sound silly, but I actually had a tear in my eye when I saw the finish line. If you get one thing out of this book, I pray it would be that you will be inspired to run across the finish line in any race.

Running has become a passion for me, and I have scheduled many events for this year, along with the ING Marathon/Half Marathon in Atlanta and a couple of triathlons. I'm willing to bet I will able to run a marathon sooner than later. From the couch to the road . . . it feels wonderful!

Chapter Two

Terms

Diet Terms

Amino Acids: A group of compounds that that serve as the building blocks from which protein and muscle are made.

Antioxidants: Small compounds that minimize tissue oxidation and help control free radicals and their negative effects.

Calorie: The unit for measuring the energy value of foods.

Carbohydrate: Organic compounds containing carbon, hydrogen, and oxygen. They are a very effective fuel source for the body. Carbohydrates contain four calories per gram.

Cholesterol: A type of fat that, although most widely known as a bad fat implicated in promoting heart disease and stroke, is a vital component in the production of many hormones in the body. There are different types of cholesterol: namely, HDL and LDL (HDL being the good form and the LDL being the bad form).

Clean Diet: This refers to eating nutrient rich, low fat meals.

Complex Carbohydrates: Foods that are high in complex carbohydrates include bread, pasta, rice, beans, vegetables and potatoes. This type of carbohydrates is made up of complex molecules and the body requires time to digest them, which means that the we fell full for a longer time period after eating.

Diet: Food and drink regularly consumed by a person, often according to specific guidelines to improve physical condition.

Essential Fatty Acids (EFAs): Fats our bodies can't make, so we must obtain them through our diets. These fats (which include linolenic acid) are very important to hormone production, as well as cellular synthesis and integrity. Good source of these fats are flaxseed oil and safflower oil.

Fat: One of the macronutrients. Fats contain nine calories per gram; it has the most calories of all the macronutrients. There are two types of fats, saturated (bad) fat and unsaturated (good) fat.

Frequent feeding: Eating often throughout the day to work with your body, not against it. By eating more often throughout the day about every two hours, you can keep your metabolism up and energy high.

Glucose: the simplest sugar molecule. It's also the main sugar found in the blood and is used as a basic fuel for the body.

HDL: (High Density Lipoprotein) is one of the subcategories of cholesterol. This is thought of as the good cholesterol. It has been shown that regular exercise raises HDL levels.

LDL: (Low Density Lipoprotein) is one of the subcategories of cholesterol. This is thought of as the bad cholesterol. LDL levels can be raised by eating a lot of saturated fats and lack of exercise.

Metabolic Rate: The rate you convert energy stored into working energy.

Metabolism: The use of nutrients by the body. It's the process by which substances come into the body and the rate at which they are used.

Proteins: Are the building blocks of muscles, enzymes, and some hormones. They are made up of amino acids and are essential for growth and repair in the body. A gram of protein contains four calories. Proteins are broken up by the body to produce amino acids.

Saturated Fats: These are the bad fats. They are called saturated because they contain no open spots on their carbon skeletons. These bad fats have been shown to raise cholesterol levels in the body.

Simple Carbohydrates: (also called sugars) is simply carbohydrates that can be found in white table sugar, preservatives, candies, coke, cake, juice concentrates, honey and glucose syrup. Simple carbohydrates are made up of single or double molecules and are quickly absorbed into the blood stream.

Unsaturated Fats: These are the good fats. These are called unsaturated because they have one or more open spots on their carbon skeletons.

Training Terms

Aerobic: This means "requiring oxygen". Aerobic metabolism occurs during low intensity, long-duration exercise, like jogging.

Anaerobic: This means "without oxygen". Anaerobic metabolism in the muscle tissue occurs during intense physical activities like sprinting or weight lifting.

Anabolic Steroids: Are actually artificially produced male hormones.

Atrophy: A decrease in size or "wasting away" of muscle tissue from lack of use.

Barbell: A free weight consisting of a long bar on which weight plates are placed. It is normally lifted with both arms.

Burnout: Burnout is used to refer to the loss of enthusiasm and energy related to an activity due to over-excessive or high levels of a particular activity.

Components of Fitness: The components of fitness are the

Concentration: The lifting phase of an exercise, when the muscle shortens or contracts.

Dumbbell: A free weight made up of a short handle on which weight plates are placed.

Eccentric: The lowering phase of an exercise, when the muscle lengthens.

Fast Twitch Muscle Fiber: Fast twitch muscle fiber is a type of muscle fiber that is suited for high intensity exercise.

Over-Training: Over-training is a condition that arises due to an imbalance between training and recovery.

Plyometrics: Plyometrics is a type of training that is designed to improve both power and strength.

Resistance Training: this type of training refers to any type of training or exercise where resistance is applied to the body like running up hills or weight training.

Slow Twitch Muscle Fiber: Slow twitch muscle fibers are the muscle fibers that are designed for endurance and high aerobic activity. They can produce a large amount of energy using oxygen.

Chapter Three

No Fads Just Facts

Insulin (Sugar)

What does glucose do for you? How does sugar sabotage your diet? Let's see. Let's look closer at sugar. Glucose is used by your body for energy. In order for glucose to get to the cells it needs a transporter. This is where insulin comes in. It transports the glucose to the cells with the open receptors. Once all receptors sites in the brain, other organs and muscles are closed the insulin then takes the glucose to storage sites (fat stores).

Refined sugar is rapidly converted to glucose in the body. That's why you get a buzz or sugar high right after you eat sugar. The problem is that because there is so much sugar in the system after a sugary snack the body cannot utilize all of the glucose so the body releases more insulin to rapidly get the glucose out of the system. The easiest way for the body to do that is to shuffle the excess into fat stores quickly. That's why you crash, no energy then the body wants to get energy but the energy has already been stored.

So as you can see sugar can sabotage your diet. But as one friend tells me all the time, "you ask people to do things they can't, like throw away sugar people aren't going to follow your plan if you have such drastic changes". I agree but those are the facts don't get mad at me. The average person can't throw away sugar, I say to that, "don't settle for average". I know throwing away the sugar bowl is not that easy. Just be mindful of the sugar content in foods.

How much sugar is too much? Probably less than you are currently eating. Most sugar is hidden and the everyday person doesn't pay attention to what they eat. So hear is the fact. The 2005 Dietary Guidelines for Americans recommends no more than 8 teaspoons per day. That is based on a 2000 calorie a day diet. One can of soda has 7 1/2 teaspoons in it. If you are reading the labels that's about 32 grams. Most people drink up too three sodas a day, see where I am going with this. We drink to many high sugary drinks. Again like I tell my friend, "Don't get mad at me it's the facts". But not all sugar is created equal. I put together a list of good sugars and bad sugars.

Good Sugars:

These are sugars that you don't need to worry about. They occur naturally in foods.

Low Fat Milk
Fresh/frozen fruit (apples, blueberries, oranges, pineapples, strawberries, and bananas).
Most vegetables

Bad Sugars:
These are sugars you'll need to limit. Thus is only a small sample but you will get the idea.

Fruit loops
Low fat yogurt
Ketchup
Syrup

Foods that sound healthy, but are loaded with sugar.

Granola
Dried fruit
Beverage (Orange juice/apple juice)
Soda (Coke, Sprite)
Snapple, Lemon Iced Tea

Snacks/Deserts
Balance/Powerbar
Frozen Yogurt
Restaurant Chocolate Cake
Fast Food Vanilla Shake

Food companies seldom list sugar in the ingredients. It will usually be listed as sucrose, dextrose or some other "ose" item. Under carbohydrates, companies now have to show sugar and fiber content. If a food has 15 grams of carbohydrates per serving and 12 of those are sugar you might want to find another choice.

In conclusion don't eat simple carbohydrates (candy, sodas, sugar) eat complex carbohydrates such as fruits so that the absorption of glucose is slow, not fast where it then will go to fat cells.

Chapter Four

My Goals

Weight Loss

You must understand that weight loss will only take place when the calories expended by the body are more than the calories consumed. Therefore reducing the calories through a well balanced diet is important for most weight loss cases. The RMR (resting metabolic rate), which is the amount of calories consumed by the human body at rest while performing essential bodily functions such as beating of the heart and keeping the body warm makes a huge difference to the calories consumed by the person. The more the lean body mass (muscle weight), the more the RMR of the body. The persons lean body mass should be increased through weight training and aerobic exercise so as to increase the RMR. This is fact people can't get any easier than that. Well somewhat anyway. If it was that simple then why is America getting fat?

This is important for all of the people who used the fad diets and gained more weight after they lost weight. If the weight loss program leads to weight loss accompanied by a loss in lean body mass (not exercising), it will also mean that the RMR will reduce as well. The reduced RMR will mean the body will require less energy while at rest and the chances of regaining the weight will be extremely high. It is recommended that a balance of aerobic and weight fitness be apart of your weight loss program. It worked for me; I gained more lean muscle which in return allowed me to burn more calories while at rest. Look at it this way. Muscle burn calories not fat. The more muscle you have the more calories you burn, the more fat you have the less calories you burn. So I ask you how do you lose weight, you burn calories sounds easy.

Weight loss requires a change of eating habits, life style change as well as regular dose of exercise to burn fat. People who are grossly overweight have a great problem on their hands, so stop worrying and attack the problem with a positive mind and motivation. Willpower is an important factor in weight loss, and you must believe in yourself that weight loss possible. You must also understand that weight loss cannot take place in a couple of days. It is a hard road that will require the person to abstain from unhealthy foods.

Benefits of exercise in a weight loss program:

1. Exercise burns calories. Physical activity uses up excess calories that otherwise would be stored as fat.
2. It leads to an increase in metabolic activity. The higher our metabolic rate, the easier it is to lose weight. In this way, exercise helps to overcome the plateau effect. The BMR or basal metabolic rate refers to the rate at which you burn calories at rest.
3. It gradually reduces your fat ratio and increases your muscle ratio. Muscle cells are 8 times more metabolically active than fat cells. So the more muscle you have the less fat you have and easier it is to lose weight.
4. It helps build self confidence. Weight loss helps to improve self image and confidence.
5. Develops will power. Overwhelming evidence suggests that the best diet is a balanced low fat diet.

Weight loss through exercise and BMI

One pound of body fat is equal to 3500 calories. So to burn one pound of fat it would take you 11.5 half-hour sessions of moderate cycling per week. This may seem difficult to most (like me) so it is best to advise that you take a healthier food intake program combined with an exercise routine to help lose weight. It is very important that you emphasize a healthier food intake rather than less food (dieting). It is my opinion that most people think that they will just simply stop eating to lose weight. That is not the case. When you stop eating it triggers your body to slow your metabolism so that your body can pull from your reserve. This is also very dangerous and could cause other health issues. You can eat and lose weight. I lost almost 74 lbs in 12 weeks and I still ate all day. I will get to that method shortly.

Proper food is essential for the maintenance or restoration of health. There are six classes of food substances: carbohydrates, fats and oils, proteins, minerals, vitamins, and water. A calorie is a unit of heat used to measure body metabolism and "how fat" individual foods will make you. Let me get scientific for a moment. Technically, a calorie is the amount of heat necessary to raise the temperature of one kilogram (2.2 pounds) of water one degree Centigrade. One gram of these nutrients when burned in the body, supplies the following number of calories. 1. carbohydrate (4 calories) 2. fat (9 calories) 3. protein (4 calories) 4. alcohol (7 calories).

From the above figures, you can see that fat is a concentrated source of calories. This is why overweight people are asked to reduce their intake of fatty foods. Alcohol is also a concentrated source of calories, supplying 7 calories/gram. This is one reason that beer drinkers end up with a beer belly. I have a saying, "you are what you eat/drink". The amount of calories needed for body functions varies with age, gender, activity, and climate. Boys are usually more active than girls and require more calories. If you eat more calories per day than you use in your body, the excess is changed to fat and stored in the body. Use this saying Eat to Live Don't Live to Eat.

I want to discuss a method that was real successful to me when I lost all my weight. It is called the ZigZag method of weight loss. The zigzag approach to weight loss is considered the most scientific method as well as a technique that leads to a long term reduction of fat. The following issues must be kept in mind while understanding the zigzag method of weight loss.

1. The more the lean body mass, the more is the RMR (resting metabolic rate or the rate at which the body consumes calories at rest) and the better the capability of the body to burn fat at rest.
2. The key to weight loss is to reduce the fat and keep the lean body mass and RMR high. By doing this, the weight loss will be permanent.
3. A calorie deficit diet leads to a reduction in fat, but also a reduction in the RMR because the lean body mass is also reduced in the calorie deficit diet.

4. The problem confronting the weight loser now is how to increase the lean body mass, which requires a positive calorie balance diet.

5. The zigzag approach is a solution to reducing fat for longer periods, increasing lean body mass and the body's RMR.

Follow these steps to make your zigzag weight loss program successful.

1. Eat more times a day. Always eat at least 5 meals a day. This will ensure that your blood sugar level is controlled. Remember the section on blood sugar. It all comes together in the end. The fat will be produced in smaller amounts, cravings for food will be lesser and the body will get a regular dose of proteins throughout the day.

2. See where the calories are coming from. In each of the 5 meals, your calorie intake should come from fats, proteins and carbohydrates in the following proportion of 1:2:3. This will mean that you are getting fewer calories from fats and the carbohydrates are the body's preferred fuel source. 1 part fat, 2 parts protein and 3 parts carbohydrates.

3. Plan the meals. Plan your meals by eating in anticipation of the calories you are about to consume in the next few hours. Eat more if you are planning to exert in the coming hours and eat less if you are about to take a nap or simply sit around. I ate more in the morning because I worked out before I went to work. Then I tapered my food intake as the day went on.

Effects of zigzagging your calories downwards for weight loss:

*   The RMR of the body will be readjusted at a higher level. This means that the body will naturally burn more calories at rest.

*   The body will be able to add more lean weight (since you should be exercising along with the controlled diet).

*   The body will be able to recover from exercise and repair tissues and muscles.

*   You will get a boost from knowing that you can gorge on food while still losing weight.

Tips to Cut Down Weight

- Build muscle to cut the weight—Protein rich foods help put more distance between hunger pains. The fuller you feel before meals, the easier it is to avoid eating. This is also applicable for women. Proteins are also made up of amino acids which help you recover from hard workouts by reducing the protein breakdown within your muscles. They also increase the testosterone and growth hormones which help you loose weight by boosting muscle growth.
- Do not eat refines carbohydrates—highly refined carbohydrates such as squashes and colas and peeled potatoes are a bad idea. One reason is that they spike up the blood sugar levels, and you feel tires and hungry when the blood sugar levels come shooting down afterwards. Frying these carbohydrates is an even worse idea.
- Eat more fiber—Fiber helps to keep food from getting absorbed into the blood stream faster giving you a consistent energy supply for longer.
- Have more calcium—Calcium rich foods have fat fighting properties and adequate calcium should be consumed from food sources everyday.
- Eat more fish—Fish contains omega-3 polyunsaturated fats which help reduce inflammation throughput the body. This helps muscle recover faster from workouts. Less inflamed muscles mean a faster metabolism which helps to cut fat. You can try cod liver oil capsules if you do not like eating fish.

Some substitutions that are essential in the diet are:

If you are eating Dairy products switch to fat free diary products.
If you are eating egg whites with yellow switch to only egg whites.
If you are using salad dressing switch to oil base salad dressing.
If you use cheese switch to low fat cheese.
If you drink fizzy drinks switch to water or fresh fruit.

Nutrition and Constituents of Food

I am going to talk about the Food Guide Pyramid that was devised by the US department of agriculture. The pyramid is facts about the foods we should eat and how much, but what you are going to say as you read this is that the pyramid states the opposite of what we have been told about good foods and bad foods for example we all have been told not to eat bread and pastas but yet we are supposed to eat 6-11 servings a day. I will break each food group down and explain how they work in our everyday diet.

Breads, Cereal, Rice, Pasta Group (6-11 servings)

This group consists of the carbohydrate heavy foods and is placed at the bottom of the pyramid indicating that they should be eaten more often and should form an important part of the daily diet. The rationale behind eating more carbohydrates is also that they provide energy and require the person to eat less fat.

Vegetables (3-5 servings) and Fruit (2-4 servings)

There is no doubt that fruits and vegetables are good for the body. Fruits and vegetables help to provide the body with essential vitamins and nutrients and also ward off diseases and ailments.

Meat, Poultry, Fish, Dry Beans, Eggs and Nuts Group (2-3 servings)

This group helps to provide the body with protein. Protein helps build the body's tissue and muscles. If you want to build more muscle which I highly recommend, I recommend a person consume about 1 gram of protein per body weight a day. This was the key in helping me lose my weight.

Milk, Yogurt and Cheese Group (2-3 servings)

This group provides protein and calcium that makes the bones strong and prevents health problems related to the degeneration of bone mass.

Fats, oils and Sweets (eat sparingly)

This group should be eaten sparingly. Fat leads to heart disease and obesity. Too much sugar also leads to obesity which can later create health problems.

So you ask why are all the foods we are told not to eat on the food pyramid. This is because the food pyramid is a balanced diet; key word is balanced not over eating all these foods but eating these foods in a balanced diet. The food guide pyramid provides an excellent way to ensure that the body's nutritional requirements are fulfilled. By following the guide, an individual will receive all the daily requirements in terms of energy, proteins, vitamins and other essential nutrients.

Fat

Fat is one of the three nutrients (along with protein and carbohydrates) that supply the calories to the body. Fat provides 9 calories per gram, more than twice the number provided by carbohydrates or protein. Fat is essential for the proper functioning of the body. Fats provide the "essential" fatty acids, which are not made by the body and must be obtained from food. Linoleic acid is the most important essential fatty acid, especially for the growth and development of infants. Fatty acids provide the raw materials that help in the control of blood pressure, blood clotting, inflammation, and other body functions. Fat serves as the storage substance for the body's extra calories. It fills the fat cells (adipose tissue) that help insulate the body. Fats are also an important energy source. When the body has used up the calories from carbohydrates, which occurs after the first 20 minutes of exercise (very important what I just said), it begins to depend on the calories from fat. Healthy skin and hair are maintained by fat. Fat helps in the absorption, and transport through the bloodstream of the fat-soluble vitamins a, D, E, and K.

Saturated Fats

Saturated fats tend to be solid at room temperature. These are the biggest dietary cause of high LDL ("bad cholesterol"). When looking at a food label, pay attention to the percent of saturated fat and avoid or limit any foods that are high (for example, over 20% saturated fat). Saturated fats are found in animal products such as butter, cheese, whole milk, ice cream, cream, and fatty meats. They are also found in some vegetable oils such as coconut, palm, and palm kernel oils.

(note: most other vegetable oils contain unsaturated fat and are healthy.)

Unsaturated Fats

Unsaturated fats tend to be liquid at room temperature. These fats help to lower blood cholesterol if used in place of saturated fats. However, unsaturated fats have a lot of calories, so you still need to limit them. Unsaturated fats are two types: mono-unsaturated and polyunsaturated. Most (but not all) liquid vegetable oils are unsaturated. (The exceptions include coconut, palm, and kernel oils.)

Trans-Fatty Acids

These fats form when vegetable oil hardens (a process called hydrogenation) and can raise LDL levels. They can also lower HDL levels ("good cholesterol"). Trans-fatty acids are found in fried foods, commercial baked goods (donuts, cookies, and crackers), processed foods, and margarines.

Hydrogenated

The term hydrogenated refers to oils that harden (such as hard butter and margarine). Foods made with hydrogenated oils should be avoided because they contain high levels of trans fatty acids, which are linked to heart disease. Keep in mind when you are looking at labels that the term "hydrogenated" and "saturated" are related; oil becomes saturated when hydrogen is added.

Eating to much saturated fat is one of the major risk factors for heart disease. A diet high in saturated fat causes a soft, waxy substance called cholesterol to build up in the arteries. Too much fat also increases the risk of heart disease because of its high calorie content, which increases the chance of becoming obese (another risk factor for heart disease and some types of cancer). Reducing daily fat intake is not guaranteed against developing cancer or heart disease, but it does help reduce the risk factors. Choose lean, protein-rich foods, fish, skinless chicken, very lean meat, and fat free or 1% dairy products. Eat foods that are naturally low in fat like whole grains, fruits, and vegetables. Get plenty of soluble fiber with oats, bran, dry peas, beans, cereal, and rice.

Carbohydrates

Carbohydrates are sometimes referred to as starches, simple sugars and sugars. Carbohydrates are one of the main dietary components. This category of foods includes sugars, starches, and fiber. The primary function of carbohydrates is to provide for the body, especially the brain and the nervous system. Your liver breaks down carbohydrates into glucose (blood sugar), which is used for energy by the body. Carbohydrates are classified as simple or complex. The classification depends on the chemical structure of the particular food source and reflects how quickly the sugar is digested and absorbed. Remember in chapter three when I was talking about insulin and how it affects weight. You will get a better understanding on how the wrong carbohydrates turn into sugar.

There are three basic types of carbohydrates, simple, complex and very complex carbohydrates. Out of these the last two types are essential for healthy diet.

- Simple Carbohydrates (also called sugars): Simple carbohydrates can be found in white sugar, preservatives, candies, soda, cake, juice concentrates, honey and glucose syrup. Simple carbohydrates are made up of single or double molecules and are quickly absorbed into the blood stream.
- Complex carbohydrates: Foods that are high in complex carbohydrates include whole grain bread, pasta, rice, beans, vegetables and potatoes. This type of carbohydrate is made up of complex molecules and the body requires time to digest them, which means that we fell full for a longer time period after eaten them
- Very complex carbohydrates (also known as fiber): This type of carbohydrate adds the bulk to our food that helps in digestion, such

as found in whole meal bread and phsylum husk. Fibers help to ease the flow of food through the intestines and reduce the risk of diabetes and lowers cholesterol. 30-35 grams of fiber a day is beneficial for the body. Very complex carbohydrates have an extremely complex molecule structure.

Excessive carbohydrates can cause an increase in total caloric intake, causing obesity. While on the other hand, deficient carbohydrates can cause a lack of calories (malnutrition), or excessive intake of fats to make up the calories. For most people, between 40% and 60% of total calories should come from carbohydrates, preferable from complex carbohydrates (starches) and naturally occurring sugars that can be found in fruits. Complex carbohydrates provide calories, vitamins, minerals, and fiber. Foods that are high in processed, refined simple sugars provide calories, but they have few nutritional benefits. It is wise to limit such sugars. Wow no wonder people are confused when it comes to losing weight.

To increase complex carbohydrates and healthy nutrients:

- Eat more fruits and vegetable.
- Eat more whole grains, rice, breads, and cereals.
- Eat more legumes (beans, lentils, and dried peas).

Protein

Proteins are complex organic compounds. The basic structure of protein is a chain of amino acids. Protein is the main component of muscles, organs, and glands. Every living cell and all body fluids, except bile and urine, contain protein. The cells of muscles, tendons, and ligaments are maintained with protein. Children and adolescents require protein for growth and development. Proteins are described as essential and nonessential proteins or amino acids. The human body requires approximately 20 amino acids for the synthesis of its proteins. The body can make only 13 of the amino acids—these are known as the nonessential amino acids. They are called non-essential because the body can make them and does not need to get them from the diet. There are 9 essential amino acids that are obtained only from food, and not made in the body. If the protein in a food supplies enough of the essential amino acids, it is called a complete protein. If the protein of a food source does not supply all the essential amino acids, it is called incomplete protein.

All meat and other animal products are sources of complete proteins. These include beef, lamb, pork, poultry, fish, shell fish, eggs, milk, and milk products. A diet high in meat could lead to high cholesterol or other diseases, such as gout. Another potential problem is that high-protein diets may put a strain on the kidneys. Extra waste matter, which is the end product of protein metabolism, is excreted in the urine.

Below shows some foods and their protein and calorie content.

Protein content of some foods

One egg has six grams of protein and 80 calories.
One half serving of skinless chicken breast has 26 grams of protein and 140 calories.
Three ounces of canned tuna has 22 grams of protein and 100 calories.
Three ounces of salmon has 23 grams of protein and 180 calories.
Six large shrimp has 8.5 grams of protein and 45 calories.
One cup of low fat yogurt has 8 grams of protein and 160 calories (sugared).
One cup of skim milk has 8 grams of protein and 86 calories.
One cup of white rice has 5 grams of protein and 240 calories.
One cup of pasta has 5 grams of protein and 160 calories.
Two slices of bread has 6 grams of protein and 160 calories.
One large bagel has 10 grams of protein and 270 calories.

Not all protein found in food can be used by the body. For example, if you eat 10 grams of protein from a particular food you may only be able to use 8 grams and the rest cannot be absorbed by the body as protein.

Choose a portion of protein and carbohydrates from each column to make a meal. Add a serving of vegetables to at least two of your daily meals. So you can see that there are plenty of foods on the list to keep you happy. You can make plenty of meals from the list. Get creative and enjoy.

Proteins:

Chicken Breast

Turkey Breast

Lean ground turkey

Leans steak

Salmon

Tuna

Crab

Lobster

Shrimp

Top round steak

Lean ground beef

Egg whites Protein shakes

Carbohydrates:

Baked potato

Sweet potato

Yam

Squash Steamed brown rice

Streamed wild rice

Pasta

Oatmeal

Beans

Corn

Strawberries

Melon

Apple

Orange

Whole wheat bread

Vegetables:

Broccoli

Lettuce

Carrots Cauliflower

Green beans
Green peppers
Mushrooms
Spinach
Tomato
Peas
Cabbage
Celery
Zucchini
Onion

Since we are talking about protein I wanted to explain how important amino acids are. Amino Acids are the chemical units or "building blocks" of the body that make up proteins. As you already know protein substances make up the muscles, tendons, organs, glands, nails, and hair. Growth, repair and maintenance of all cells are dependent upon them. Next to water, protein makes up the greatest portion of your body weight. Amino Acids that must be obtained from the diet are called "Essential Amino Acids" other Amino Acids that the body can manufacture from other sources are called "NonEssential Amino Acids."

Histidine (Essential Amino Acids)

Is found abundantly in hemoglobin; has been used in the treatment of rheumatoid arthritis, allergies, ulcers and anemia; is essential for the growth and repair of tissues; important for the maintenance of the myelin sheaths, which protect nerve cells; is needed for the production of both red and white blood cells; protects the body from radiation damage; lowers blood pressure, aids in the removal of heavy metals from the body; aids in sexual arousal.

Isoleucine (Essential Amino Acid)

Is needed for hemoglobin formation; stabilizes and regulates blood sugar and energy levels; is valuble to athletes because it aids in the healing and repair of muscle tissue, skin and bones; has been found to be deficient in people suffering from certain mental and physical disorders.

Leucine (Essential Amino Acid)

Works with Isoleucine and Valine to promote the healing of muscle tissue, skin, and bones; is recommended for those recovering from surgery; lowers blood sugar levels; aids in increasing growth hormone production.

Lysine (Essential Amino Acid)

Ensures adequate calcium absorption and maintains a proper nitrogen balance in adults; helps form collagen (which makes up cartilage and connective tissue); aids in the production of antibodies which have the ability to fight cold sores and herpes outbreaks; lowers high serum triglyceride levels.

Methionine (Essential Amino Acid)

A powerful anti-oxidant and a good source of sulfur, which prevents disorders of the hair, skin, and nails; assist the breakdown of fats, thus helping to prevent a buildup of fat in the liver and arteries, that might obstruct blood flow to the brain, heart, and kidneys; helps to detoxify harmful agents such as lead and other heavy metals; helps diminish muscle weakness; prevents brittle hair; protects against the affects of radiation; beneficial for women who take oral contraceptives because it promotes the excretion of estrogen; reduces the levels of histamine in the body which can cause the brain to relay wrong messages; helpful to individuals suffering from schixophrenia.

Phenylalanine (Essential Amino Acid)

Used by the brain to produce norepinephrine, a chemical that transmits signals between nerve cells in the brain; promotes alertness and vitality; elevates mood; decreases pain; aids in memory and learning; used to treat arthritis; depression,menstral cramps, migraines, obesity, Parkinson's disease, and schizophrenia.

Threonine (Essential Amino Acid)

Helps maintain proper protein balance in the body; is important for the formation of collagen, elastin and tooth enamel; aids liver and Lipotropic function when combined with Aspartic Acid and Methionine; prevents the buildup of fat in the liver; assists; assists metabolism and assimilation.

Tryptophan (Essential Amino Acid)

A natural relaxant, helps alleviate insomnia by inducing normal sleep; reduces anxiety and depression and stabilizes mood; helps in the treatment of migraine headaches; helps the immune system function properly; aids in weight control by reducing appetite; enhances the release of growth hormones; helps control hyperactivity in children.

Valine (Essential Amino Acid)

Is needed for muscle metabolism and coordination, tissue repair, and for the maintenance of proper nitrogen balance in the body; used as an energy source by muscle tissue; helpful in treating liver and gallbladder disease; promotes mental vigor and calm emotions.

Alanine (Non-Essential Amino Acid)

Plays a major role in the transfer of nitrogen from peripheral tissue to the liver; aids in the metabolism of glucose, a simple carbohydrate that the body uses for energy; guards against the buildup of toxic substances that are released into the muscle cells when muscle protein is broken down quickly to meet energy needs, such as what happens with aerobic exercise; strengthens the immune system by producing antibodies.

Arginine (Non-Essential Amino Acid)

Considered "The Natural Viagra" by increasing blood flow to the penis; retards the growth of tumors and cancer by enhancing the immune system; increases the size and activity of the thymus gland, which manufactures T cells, crucial components of the immune system; aids in liver detoxification by neutralizing ammonia, reduces the effects of chronic alcohol toxicity; used in treating sterility in men by increasing sperm count; aids in weight loss because it facilitates an increase in muscle mass and reduction of body fat; assists the release of growth hormones, which is crucial for "optimal" muscle growth and tissue repair; is a major component of collagen which is good for arthritis and connective tissue disorders; aids in stimulating the pancreas to release insulin.

Aspartic Acid (Non-Essential Amino Acid)

Increases stamina and is good for cronic fatigue and depression; rejuvenates cellular activity, cell formation and metabolism, which gives you a younger looking appearance; protects the liver by aiding the expulsion of ammonia; combines with other amino acids to form molecules that absorb toxins and remove them from the bloodstream; helps facilitate the movement of certain minerals across the intestinal lining and into the blood and cells; aids the function of RNA and DNA, which are carriers of genetic information.

Cysteine & Cystine (Non-Essential Amino Acid)

Functions as a powerful anti-oxidant in detoxifying harmful toxins; protects the body from radiation damage; protects the liver and brain from damage due to alcohol, drugs, and toxic compounds found in cigarette smoke; has been used to treat rheumatoid arthritis and hardening of the arteries; promotes the recovery from severe burns and surgery; promotes the burning of fat and the building of muscle; slows down the aging process. Skin and hair is made up of 10-14% Cystine.

Glutamic Acid (Non-Essential Amino Acid)

Is an excitatory neurotransmitter for the central nervous system, the brain and spinal cord; important in the metabolism of sugars and fats; aids in the transportation of potassium into the spinal fluid; acts as fuel for the brain; helps correct personality disorders, and is used in the treatment of epilepsy, mental retardation, muscular dystrophy, and ulcers.

Glutamine (Non-Essential Amino Acid)

The most abundant amino acid found in the muscle; helps build and maintain muscle tissue; helps prevent muscle wasting that can accompany prolonged bed rest or diseases such as cancer and AIDS; a "brain fuel" that increases brain function and mental activity; assists in maintaining the proper acid/alkaline balance in the body; promotes a healthy digestive tract; shortens the healing time of ulcers and alleviates fatigue, depression and impotence; decreases sugar cravings and the desire for alcohol; recently used in the treatment of schizophrenia and senility.

Glycine (Non-Essential Amino Acid)

Retards muscle degeneration; improves glycogen storage, thus freeing up glucose for energy needs; promotes a healthy prostate, central nervous system, and immune system; useful for repairing damaged tissue and promotes healing.

Ornithine (Non-Essential Amino Acid)

Helps to prompt the release of growth hormones, which promotes the metabolism of excess body fat (this effect is enhanced if combined with Arginine and Carnitine; is necessary for a healthy immune system; detoxifies ammonia and aids in liver regeneration; stimulates insulin secretion and helps insulin work as an anabolic (muscle building) hormone.

Proline (Non-Essential Amino Acid)

Improves skin texture by aiding the production of collagen and reducing the loss of collagen through the aging process; helps in the healing and the strengthening of joints, tendons, and heart muscle, works with Vitamin C to promote healthy connective tissue.

Serine (Non-Essential Amino Acid)

Needed for the proper metabolism of fats and fatty acids, the growth of muscle, and the maintenance of healthy immune system; is a component of the protective myelin sheaths that cover nerve fibers; is important in RNA & DNA function and cell formation; aids in the production of immunoglobulins and antibodies.

Taurine (Non-Essential Amino Acid)

Strengthens the heart muscle, boosts vision, and helps prevent muscular degeneration; is the key component of bile, which is needed for the digestion of fats; useful for people with atherosclerosis, edema, heart disorders, hypertension, or hypoglycemia; is vital for the proper utilization of sodium, potassium, calcium and magnesium; helps prevent the development of potentially dangerous cardiac arrhythmias; has been used to treat anxiety, epilepsy, hyperactivity, poor brain function, and seizures.

Tyrosine (Non-Essential Amino Acid)

Is important to overall metabolism; is a precursor of adrenaline, nor epinephrine, and dopamine, which regulate mood and stimulates metabolism and the nervous system; acts as a mood elevator, suppresses the appetite, helps reduce body fat; aids in the production of melanin 9the pigment responsible for hair and skin color) and in the functions of the adrenal, thyroid, and pituitary glands; has been used to help chronic fatigue, narcolepsy, anxiety, depression, low sex drive, allergies and headaches.

The Human Digestive System

Since we are talking about weight loss and diet I wanted to add a section in the book to explain how the digestive system works. After you eat your food is used and broken down into nutrients for the body. You need to know how your food is turned into the fuel and nutrients your body needs. So often, we eat things that have no benefit to our body.

Digestion in the stomach—The stomach has flexible walls and can accommodate and store a large amount of food. This allows for the food to be released from the stomach at regular intervals to the rest of the alimentary canal. The lining of the stomach produces gastric juices containing the enzyme pepsin. Pepsin acts on the protein in the food and breaks it down into soluble compounds called peptides. The stomach wall also secretes hydrochloric acid which makes a diluted acid mixture in the stomach. The acid provides an atmosphere for the pepsin to work on the food and also helps to kill the bacteria in the food. The stomach churns up the food every 20 seconds through a rhythmic motion. The amount of time that food remains in the stomach may vary greatly from a few minutes in the case of water to 1-2 hours in the case of fats and proteins.

Digestion in the small intestine—The food mixed with acid and saliva moves from the stomach to the small intestine. An alkaline juice from the pancreas and bile from the liver are poured over the food. This happens in the upper area of the small intestine called the duodenum. The juice from the pancreas contains enzymes that act on carbohydrates, proteins and fats. Proteins are broken down into soluble amino acids, starch is broken down into maltose and fats are split up into fatty acids and glycerol. Bile helps to digest fats. The food moves on to the lower part of the small intestine called the ileum where further enzymes are the secreted to convert the unchanged proteins to amino acids, maltose and other sugars to glucose and unchanged fats to fatty acids and glycerol. Nearly all the absorption of undigested food takes place in the ileum as well. Small hair like projections in the ileum called villi absorb molecules of the digested food (mainly amino acids and glucose) and it enters the blood stream through the dense network of small blood vessels in the villi.

Digestion in the large intestine—The material passing into the large intestine largely consists of water and undigested matter (mostly cellulose, vegetable matter and other roughage), dead cells, and bacteria. The large intestine does not secrete any enzyme and can absorb very little digested food.

Storage of glucose in digested food takes place when the quantity of food is in excess of the amount required by the body. Glucose is required in the blood for generating energy. If a person has not eaten for 8 hours, the blood sugar level would hover around 90-100mg/100 cm3 of blood. After a meal containing carbohydrates the blood sugar level may raise to about 140mg/100cm3, but 2 hours later the level will come down again to about 95mg. The sugar that is not immediately required for producing energy is converted into glycogen in the liver and muscles. The glycogen molecule is built up by combining many glucose molecules. About 100 grams of this insoluble glycogen is stored in the liver and about 300 grams in the muscles. When the sugar level falls below 80 mg/100cm3, the liver converts its glycogen back to glucose for energy production. The muscle glycogen is used as a source of energy for the muscles just like glucose. The glycogen in the liver is a short term store, about 6 hours if no other glucose supply is available. Ok listen excess glucose, not stored as glycogen is converted into fat deposits in the body. So that is why you should not consume an abundant amount of sugar.

Fat and how it enters your body

The basics of body fat in the human body contain two types of fat tissue. White fat is important in energy metabolism, heat insulation and mechanical cushioning. Brown fat is found mostly in newborn babies. Adults have little to no brown fat so I won't concentrate on it.

Fat tissue is made up of fat cells, which are a unique type of cell. You can think of a fat cell as a tiny plastic bag that holds a drop of fat. White fat cells are large cells that have very little cytoplasm, only 15 percent cell volume, a small nucleus and one large fat droplet that makes up 85 percent of cell volume.

Fat enters your body when you eat food that contains fat, mostly triglycerides, it goes through your stomach and intestines. In the intestines, the following happens:

1. Large fat droplets get mixed with bile salts from the gall bladder in a process called emulsification. The mixture breaks up the large droplets into several smaller droplets called micelles, increasing the fat's surface area.

2. The pancreas secretes enzymes called lipases that attack the surface of each micelle and break the fats down into their parts, glycerol and fatty acids.

3. These parts get absorbed into the cells lining the intestine.

4. In the intestine cell, these parts are reassembled into packages of fat molecules (triglycerides) with a protein coating called chylomicrons. The protein coating makes the fat dissolve more easily in water.

5. The chylomicrons are released into the lymphatic system—they do not go directly into the bloodstream because they are too big to pass through the wall of the capillary.

6. The lymphatic system eventually merges with the veins, at which point the cylomicrons pass into the bloodstream.

Insulin and fat storage

When you eat a candy bar or a meal, the presence of glucose, amino acids or fatty acids in the intestine stimulates the pancreas to secrete a hormone called insulin. Insulin acts on many cells in your body, especially those in the liver, muscle and fat tissue. Insulin tells the cells to do the following:

- Absorb glucose, fatty acids and amino acids
- Stop breaking down:

    A. Glucose, fatty acids and amino acids
    B. Glycogen into glucose
    C. Fats into fatty acids and glycerol
    D. Proteins into amino acids

- Start building:

    A. Glycogen from glucose
    B. Fats (triglycerides) from glycerol and fatty acids
    C. Proteins from amino acids

The activity of lipoprotein lipases depends upon the levels of insulin in the body. If insulin is high, then the lipases are highly active; if insulin is low, the lipases are inactive.

The fatty acids are then absorbed from the blood into fat cells, muscle cells and liver cells. In these cells, under stimulation by insulin, fatty acids are made into fat molecules and stored as fat droplets.

It is also possible for fat cells to take up glucose and amino acids, which have been absorbed into the blood stream after a meal, and convert those into fat molecules. The conversion of carbohydrates or protein into fat is 10 times less efficient than simply storing fat in a fat cell, but the body can do it. If you have 100 extra calories in fat (about 11 grams) floating in your blood stream, fat cells can store it using only 2.5 calories of energy. On the other hand, if you have 100 extra calories in glucose (about 25 grams) floating in your bloodstream, it takes 23 calories of energy to convert the glucose into fat and then store it. Given a choice, a fat cell will grab the fat and store it rather than the carbohydrates because fat is so much easier to store. So my advice is reducing your fat intake.

Stay with me I know this all sounds boring but I am going to get to the part where it helps you to understand how to lose weight. Braking down body fat and losing weight and losing fat.

Fad Diets

Americans are obsessed with dieting. We always try the latest diets appearing in popular magazines, talk shows and commercials late at night. Many fad diets defy logic, basic biochemistry, and even appetite appeal. They are popular because they promise quick results with no exercise. We have just gotten plain lazy no other way to say it.

Unfortunately the one thing most fad diets have in common is that they seldom promote sound weight loss. More important, they only work short-term. As many as 95% of people who lose weight with fad diets gain it back within five years but you have already paid good money for that diet. Then you pay more money for another diet because the one you used four years ago is already outdated like a computer.

Despite the popularity of dieting obesity has increased steadily since the 70's. In the 80's 25% of adults in the United States were overweight. By 1991, this figure had risen to 33%, and by 2001, over 66% of the adult population were classified as overweight or obese. Each year, Americans spend more than $30 billion fighting fat, often for gimmicks that do not work. Most of you trying to lose weight are not using the recommended combination of reduced caloric intake and increasing physical activity.

Knowledgeable practitioners do not recommend fad diets because such diets do not work long-term. Even though they might work in the short run, there is little value in losing weight if one is only going to regain it after the diet ends. With repeated dieting, weight loss becomes more difficult and results in frustration, feeling of failure, and loss of self-esteem.

From a nutritional standpoint, many fad diets lack important nutrients. For example, high-fat, low-carbohydrate diets are low in vitamins E, A, thiamine, B6, folate, calcium, magnesium, iron, zinc, potassium, and dietary fiber, and also require supplementation. In addition, they are high in saturated fat and cholesterol. When individuals are allowed to choose foods from all the food groups, their diet is likely to be nutritionally adequate and healthier long-term.

Keep this in mind; there are no magic bullets when it comes to healthy weight loss. No matter which marketing phrase a fad diet uses, it isn't reasonable to expect miraculous weight loss that will last. The trick is to find an everyday eating plan that not only keeps the pounds off but also provides the right balance of calories and nutrition and also exercise and that combination requires a lifestyle change. Can you commit to that if so you will succeed in weight loss? We will get to that later in the book.

You'll know it's a fad diet if it:

- Promises magic or miracle foods that burn fat.
- Requires you to eat unusual quantities of only one food or food types.
- Requires rigid menus of a limited selection of foods to be eaten at a specific time and day.
- Requires you to eat specific food combinations in a certain sequences or combinations.
- Promises rapid weight loss of more than two pounds a week.
- Has no warning for those with diabetes or high blood pressure to seek medical advice before starting the diet.
- Does not include increased physical activity as part of the plan.

You may have tried over and over again to lose weight, but with none or little success. There's no point feeling bad or disappointed, the truth is losing weight is not easy. No magic pill that will melt away extra pounds and keep them off. Let me be blunt about it, fad diets don't work and with all the commercials out their promising miracle no wonder we all are confused. I am not offering you a magic pill either with this book, just the right tools to get you on your way to a lifestyle change.

I was 236lbs of fat that had an unhealthy control of my everyday life. I had limits to everyday task. It was when I was out to play with my kids and found myself stopping after a few minutes to catch my breath. I decided then that I needed to change. I set goals that would last for a lifetime. I will be competing in 5k's, 10'ks and marathons. The feeling of completing what you started is self gratifying. Remember most exercise plans work we just don't stick with it long enough to see the results.

Running

Before when you mention the word running I would get sick to my stomach. I never really went in to this with a goal to compete in any running event. I know I said in the beginning that one of my goals was to start and finish a 5k, but when I ran in the Firecracker 5k in Shreveport and made it in 33:30 I was hooked. The race was in July and anyone living in Louisiana knows in July it's down right hot. I remember getting to the event almost an hour early. I was so nervous my heart was about to jump out. Start and finish that's what I kept saying over and over and the gun fired. At this time I had already lost about 65lbs so my weight wasn't a factor. I think my problem was I did not want to come in last. Who wants to be the last to cross? One mile in I see a huge hill, o know I did not prepare for this but going up the hill did not bother me it was when I started to go down that slowed me down. As I got to around mile three I looked back and saw that I was in the middle of the pack and I was not winded and from there I never stopped and not only finished my first 5k but did not finish last.

Seeing the crowd that cheered everyone on to finish the race was a spectacular sight. The support was extremely showcased throughout the race. From that point on I was hooked and a year and a half later I have ran in many 5ks, training to compete in triathlons and in March 2008 competed in the ING Half Marathon in Atlanta.

As I set in my hotel room on the 10th floor in down town Atlanta the night before the big race I lay quietly looking out the window at rain. I can feel my heart pounding not nervously but excited. I go over the track over and over again. The local news has highlights from last year's race on the TV. I look over at the clock as the hours start to go by. I need to sleep but I am too excited. It is 12:30 am and I have a wake up call at 5:30am. Finally I look out the window one more time and see that the rain has stopped.

Morning is finally here; I get up take a shower and go down to the lobby for a bite of fruit with some of the other runners. I can see it in their eyes how they feel. Like a duck on the pond. I like to use that phrase when I am nervous but I don't want anyone to know. You know like a duck, it is calm and still on the surface but under the water there feet are moving frantically. We all leave together to go to the staging area. The Olympic runners are already their warming up. The Kenyans are jogging around the practice area to loosen up. Before the race you have to get your chip programmed in so that you can be followed during the race. I stepped on the mat 45 minutes before the gun went off at 7:00am.

The weather was supposed to be nice with temperature at the start off the race around 50 degrees and warming up to around 70 degrees before the end of the race. The actual temperature at the start was around 39 degrees and it never reached 45 degrees during the race. It had a cold misty rain in the air that I noticed did not affect the runners. The professionals went off first as they averaged a record breaking stride. I remember stopping when they made their way to pass use at the turn. I had never been so amazed at the talent that just passed inches from me. These guys are going to run in the Olympics and other professional races around the world. The first Olympian was a Russian by the name of Oleg Marusin. He never broke stride as he passed us on a steep incline that did not recede for about a half a mile. That was the first time in the race that I saw a motor cycle escort. Right behind him was a Kenyan that everyone kept talking about, Jonathan Ndambuki. Again he brushed by me barley touching my shoulder but he was moving so fast I could not say sorry.

The woman had a strong showing also with Alena Vinitskaya of the country Belarus. She beat last year's winner by 12 seconds. All of these athletes have my respect because until you try one you really don't know how hard it is to compete in a race of this magnitude with the weather conditions and hills.

As for myself I was so pumped when the starting gun fired. By the time I could catch my breath I had already ran 4 miles. My adrenaline was pumping so high it carried me for the first 6 miles. By mile seven you can start to notice the distance from each person. By this time you can start passing more easily. I remember at times I would catch myself in the moment looking around at the buildings in the back ground, listening to others trying to encourage their friends that ran with them. The crowd on the side of the streets yelling at all of us. It was like a parade and I was in it. Magazine photographers lined throughout the track taken pictures of the event. Just breathe taking at the whole experience. I could probably catch a tear in my eyes on occasion.

Coming up to the last couple of miles I started noticing my legs starting to hurt. Not a cramp but hurting a little. Hoping no more hills from this point ahead I tried to think of the finish line. I think the hills finally got to my legs towards the end. As we came up to another hydration station I hear someone say almost there you only have two more miles left. When I heard that my adrenaline kicked in like it did at the beginning of the race. The last mile I came to my last hill. It was not as big as the others but it was close. I can see at the bottom the finish line with cameras flashing and video vans filming. The last quarter mile they have you run right in front of the camera so they can get your picture coming across the finish line. As I start the last fifty yards thousands of spectators are yelling at you encouraging you to finish and has I stepped across the line and an official hugs you with your medal you can't help but to brake down because I had just finished the hardest thing I had ever done. My time in the half marathon was 2:43:18. My goal was to finish under four hours.

By far the ING Marathon/Half Marathon was the most exciting thing I have accomplished since I lost my weight. I am already scheduled to run in the Chevron Half Marathon in January 2009 and will be back at the ING Marathon in Atlanta to run in the full Marathon. I also have taken part in triathlons which I will be in the Iron Man event in New Orleans April 2009.

I want to say a special thank you to two friends of mine that if not for their wonderful talent putting this book together would have been very hard. And, I want to thank YMCA of Baton Rouge for allowing me to use their facility.

Edited by Tanya Parrish. Thank you so much for putting my words on paper so that all can enjoy. Your soft and special voice is a blessing the Lord gave you to help me.

Author photo by Candi Shaffer again the Lord gave you a wonderful talent that shines through your camera.

www.ingramcontent.com/pod-product-compliance
Lightning Source LLC
Chambersburg PA
CBHW061224280526
45784CB00006B/2617